Ülvan Özad

Cartilage and Engineering

Ülvan Özad

Cartilage and Engineering

LAP LAMBERT Academic Publishing

Impressum / Imprint

Bibliografische Information der Deutschen Nationalbibliothek: Die Deutsche Nationalbibliothek verzeichnet diese Publikation in der Deutschen Nationalbibliografie; detaillierte bibliografische Daten sind im Internet über http://dnb.d-nb.de abrufbar.

Alle in diesem Buch genannten Marken und Produktnamen unterliegen warenzeichen-, marken- oder patentrechtlichem Schutz bzw. sind Warenzeichen oder eingetragene Warenzeichen der jeweiligen Inhaber. Die Wiedergabe von Marken, Produktnamen, Gebrauchsnamen, Handelsnamen, Warenbezeichnungen u.s.w. in diesem Werk berechtigt auch ohne besondere Kennzeichnung nicht zu der Annahme, dass solche Namen im Sinne der Warenzeichen- und Markenschutzgesetzgebung als frei zu betrachten wären und daher von jedermann benutzt werden dürften.

Bibliographic information published by the Deutsche Nationalbibliothek: The Deutsche Nationalbibliothek lists this publication in the Deutsche Nationalbibliografie; detailed bibliographic data are available in the Internet at http://dnb.d-nb.de.

Any brand names and product names mentioned in this book are subject to trademark, brand or patent protection and are trademarks or registered trademarks of their respective holders. The use of brand names, product names, common names, trade names, product descriptions etc. even without a particular marking in this works is in no way to be construed to mean that such names may be regarded as unrestricted in respect of trademark and brand protection legislation and could thus be used by anyone.

Coverbild / Cover image: www.ingimage.com

Verlag / Publisher:
LAP LAMBERT Academic Publishing
ist ein Imprint der / is a trademark of
OmniScriptum GmbH & Co. KG
Heinrich-Böcking-Str. 6-8, 66121 Saarbrücken, Deutschland / Germany
Email: info@lap-publishing.com

Herstellung: siehe letzte Seite /
Printed at: see last page
ISBN: 978-3-659-55408-7

Table of Contents

I would like to dedicate this book to the amazing person who taught me almost everything I know in life, my mother…

Structure and Characteristics of Cartilage and Scaffolds

Cartilage is a tough but flexible tissue providing rigidity to the structures that it supports. There are three types of cartilage: hyaline, elastic and fibrocartilage. Elastic cartilage is present in the areas needing strength, and involves elastic fibres facilitating stretching. Fibrocartilage is prevalent in the areas exposed to pressure such as intervertebral discs and has thick fibres of collagen (Tortora and Derrickson, 2006, p126-130).

The most abundant cartilage in body is hyaline cartilage which is surrounded by perichondrium membrane. It contains large amounts of fine collagen fibres and a small amount of chondrocytes (1-10%) (Marieb and Hoehn, 2009, p131-133).

It operates as articular cartilage at the joints of long bones and functions as a compression absorber. 4 zones are present in the articular cartilage. Superficial layer, with flat cells and parallel collagen arrangement has the highest collagen and lowest proteoglycan content. Transitional layer involves spherical cells and it is mainly made up of proteoglycans. Deep radial layer has arrangement of chondrocytes and collagen fibres parallel to the articular surface. The calcified cartilage layer distinguishes hyaline cartilage and subchondral bone (Wheeless, 2011). Collagen is the main constituent of the articular cartilage. Epiphyseal plates, during growth are also hyaline cartilage. Hyaline cartilage is important for compressive stress resistance of especially articulating joints (Marieb and Hoehn, 2009, p131-133).

Since the blood and nervous supplies are absent, nutrients are received by diffusion from the perichondrium. For this reason, growth and repair of cartilage are slow processes. The proliferation mainly happens in the superficial and deep calcified zones (Blitterswijk et al., 2005, p539). Interstitial growth is performed by chondrocyte division and extracellular matrix (ECM) production resulting in the chondrocytes getting further away and cartilage expanding in size. Appositional growth is mainly due to fibroblast division and differentiation into chondroblasts (Tortora and Derrickson, 2006, p129-130).

Chondroblasts are present in the areas of cartilage growth and secrete matrix which includes type 2 collagen and ground substance. Large quantities of collagen, proteoglycans such as chondroitin sulphate and keratan sulphate are present in the ground substance of cartilage. Non-aggregating and aggregating proteoglycans are present. Glycosaminoglycans (GAGs) which are found in articular cartilage are side chains of non-aggregating proteoglycans (Blitterswijk et al., 2005, p537).

Chondrocytes, the mature form of cartilage cells, are grouped in lacunae cavities due to firm structure of cartilage not allowing spreading out. ECM is very important for regulation of the mechanical characteristics of articular cartilage required for healthy functioning.

The synthesis of ECM by chondrocytes is regulated by mechanical loading (Grodzinsky et al., 2000, p691-713). Conversion of these mechanical stimuli to biological response inside cells is not completely understood. Nearly 80% of the cartilage matrix is water resulting in the presence of vast amounts of tissue fluid (Marieb and Hoehn, 2009, p131-133).

Movement of tissue fluid helps rebounding after compression together with nourishment of the cells. Type 2 collagen present in the ECM assists the resistance to tension. Small amount of proteoglycans present are important for the flow of solutes. The matrix between chondrocytes is called interterritorial ECM (Kuhnel et al., 2003, p193).

In osteoarthritis, there is deformation of cartilage resulting in catabolism of the cartilage tissue and the damaged cartilage cannot heal under normal conditions. There are various cartilage repair techniques such as debridement, marrow stimulation (Behrens, 2005, p193–197), stem cell transplants, autografts or allografts and autologous chondrocyte implantation (Saw et al., 2011, p493-506).

Tissue engineering, in order to find a treatment for this condition, is interested in artificial induction of the repair process by isolating, expanding and stimulating growth of chondrocytes in bioreactor systems followed by implantation to body (Chowdhury, 2011c).

In vitro cell division of chondrocytes decreases with age and monolayer growth results in dedifferentiation together with loss of re-differentiation ability and phenotype (Benya et al., 1982, p215-224). The studies conducted provide carrying results for protective monolayer culture outcomes according to the compression characteristics such as increase in gene expression (Das et al., 1997, p87–93).

Growth factors such as TGFβ1 and FGF-2 increase proliferation of cells and conserve the re-differentiation ability of the cells in a three dimensional environment (Blitterswijk et al., 2005, p541-543). Three-dimensional environment, however, cannot imitate the real loading conditions (Chowdhury et al., 2011).

The ideal scaffold needs to allow cell growth and should be able to permit reproduction in three-dimensional structures. Its degradation should not create toxicity and should match the tissue regeneration rate. High porosity is also required to create space for ECM production (Freed et al., 1994) and allow nutrient transport.

Three-dimensional organization is important for ECM synthesis stimulation and for prevention of phenotype loss required for the functioning of cartilage (Blitterswijk et al., 2005, p548). The disadvantage is the decreased transport of nutrients to the core resulting in decreased viability (Heywood, 2005), mainly caused by non-homogenous cell density, thickness and permeability (Choudhury, 2011).

In the case of improved homogenous distribution, nutrients would be transferred to core easily; however, oxygen and glucose utilization are important and they need to be monitored but chondrocytes are mainly anaerobic so glucose is the main important molecule, oxygen gains importance when glucose is not available since chondrocytes start performing oxidative respiration (Heywood, 2006). In the same way, increased oxygen supply could damage the cells.

6

By application of mechanical forces to three-dimensional constructs at different levels, the mechanosensitive cells such as chondrocytes respond by altering cell metabolism, by increasing the ECM synthesis and cell proliferation or by increasing damage and deformation (Parkkinjen, 1992, p610-620; Knight, 2002, p1-8) through modified signalling pathways (Chowdhury et al., 2001, p1168-1174).

A5β1 integrin is the major receptor for signalling pathway activation from the mechanical stimuli. Abnormal compressive loading in normal physiological conditions or normal compressive loading in abnormal physiology can lead to cartilage tissue damage (Chowdhury, 2011c). There are various parameters involved in this process such as the model systems used and forms of force applied.

Development of Cartilage Tissue Engineering

Failure of a specific tissue in body due to pathological, degenerative, iatrogenic or other causes could lead to serious problems for the patient. Prostheses, surgery, medications or other medical devices could be used; however, cannot treat the condition permanently (Nature Biotechnology, 2000) whereas tissue engineering aims a permanent solution through regeneration.

Tissue engineering was initiated by Hooke identifying cells in his studies (Hooke, 1665) followed by Schleiden and Schwann describing the cell theory (Schleiden, 1838, p136-178; Schwann, 1839). Loeb suggested in-vitro cell growing (Loeb, 1897). Rous and Jones commenced cell expansion by finding the role of trypsin in cell separation (Rous and Jones, 1916, p549-555). Cell extraction with techniques like centrifugation followed by trypsin or collagenase digestion provided a route for in vitro cell proliferation.

Various cell types could be used as a source such as autologous, allogenic, primary or secondary, and stem cells. Although obtaining the cells were easy, culture period added a fibrous nature to chondrocytes diminishing their required functions (Captan et al., 1997).

Since the late 90s, differentiation of embryonic and adult stem cells are under interest (Amit et al., 2000, p271-278; Winterswijk and Nout, 2007). Deep cartilage defects were repaired by mesenchymal stem cells replacing the hyaline cartilage (Caplan et al., 1997) and new hyaline cartilage tissue formed demonstrated reduced strength. Micro fractures could be created resulting in migration and differentiation of precursors in partial-thickness cartilage defects (Kim et al., 1991, p1301-1315).

The amount of chondrocyte in the body is limited and chondrocytes have species-dependent geometry (Stoltz, 2000) so using stem cells should be preferred in the future product designs.

Matrix is important; matrix implantation is needed (Buckwalter and Mankin, 1998) and scaffolds could be used for this. Due to the limited availability of natural biomaterials, synthetic scaffolds gained interest and would be favourable in mass production of new products. Growth factors either injected or formed by genetic modification (Boyan et al., 1999) or corticosteroids could improve the healing process (Schulz and Bader, 2007).

Use of scaffolds rather than periosteal grafts was an improvement because of decreased dedifferentiation, cell morbidity and anchoring that was present in two dimensional constructs (Kim and Han, 2000). Three dimensional grafts have benefits like improved biochemical conditions and phenotype, superior mechanical features, easier recovery, enhanced nutrient delivery and better surgical handling which makes them favourable for use in new products.

Disadvantages are low availability of chondrocytes and difficult proliferation (Schulz and Bader, 2007). Biodegradability is significant because scaffold needs to degrade as the new tissue forms. There have been various synthesis techniques of the scaffolds used such as electro spinning, emulsification and computer assisted design that are successfully used (Elisseeff and Ma, 2005).

Avascularity of cartilage prevents chondrocyte migration and healing so additional measures are used to promote repair (Hunziker, 2002). Mosaicplasty (osteoarticular transfer system) aims replacement of the damaged knee cartilage with many small and Osteochondral Autograft Transfer with several larger cartilage plugs from non-weight-bearing areas of knee (Hangody et al., 1998, p751-756).

Tissue engineered cartilage repair, autologous cell transplantation (ACT) or autologous cell implantation (ACI) (Kim and Han, 2000; Brittberg et al., 1994, p889-895) is the most prevalent application of the tissue engineered chondrocytes. ACI takes place by chondrocyte injection to the damaged area followed by periosteal graft (Chowdhury, 2011; Hausser and Fussenegger 2007).

Classical, matrix induced and artificial cover techniques are all used nowadays. There are ACI products in tissue engineering aiming treatment of various traumatic and degenerative conditions. Development of this technique by using stem cells, to areas other than knee or weight-bearing joints and to places involving bone and cartilage aiming all age groups and non-traumatic conditions could increase the sales (Husing et al., 2003).

Bioreactors are being used for fast and economic chondrocyte growth. The biological and mechanical factors affecting chondrocyte environment, structure and contents is important for creating and monitoring an optimum human body simulation with even nutrient distribution for cell viability (Schulz and Bader, 2007). Producing a bioreactor with efficient transportation and mechanical stimuli would improve chondrocyte growth in the new products. Cell selection, scaffold design and in-vivo stimulation are the three important elements of cartilage tissue engineering which still needs to be improved (Kuo et al., 2006, p64).

The Cell-Agarose Model and Bioreactors

In the cell-agarose model, isolated chondrocytes are embedded into agarose followed by application of compressive load in order to stimulate ECM production. This model is successful in maintaining the normal pathways for mechanotransduction and ECM synthesis (Chowdhury et al., 2003, p105-111).

Easy set up and replication, preservation of chondrocyte appearances together with adoption of spherical morphology, accessibility of variable levels of strain application and easiness in investing signalling pathways change make this model desirable.

Only disadvantage is the loss of matrix interactions which could alter the mechanosignalling (Chowdhury, 2011). The effect of compression on chondrocyte-agarose constructs varies with loading type. In terms of proteoglycan synthesis and proliferation of cells, static loading has an inhibitory effect whereas dynamic compression had a stimulatory effect (Buschmann et al., 1995, p1497–1508). One important consideration in this process is the variability of the chondrocyte response within the different sub-populations.

Glycosaminoglycans, produced by chondrocytes, are side chains of proteoglycans which are one of the major components of ECM. Increase in GAG amount also demonstrates an increase in ECM production.

The sizes of the pores are also important for nutrient transfer. Larger pores permit nutrient transfer to chondrocytes. In higher concentrations of agarose, the smaller pore radius will prevent nutrient passage to the central areas.

For mechanical properties, frequency was found to be important for proteoglycan synthesis but not for cell proliferation (Lee and Bader, 1997, p181-188). Dynamic compression can receive different responses from chondrocyte zonal sub-populations. Superficial cells respond to 1 Hz dynamic compression by increasing the cell proliferation mediated by nitric oxide down-regulation (Murrell, 1995, p15–21) and calcium; and, deep cells respond by increasing the proteoglycan synthesis (Lee et al., 1998, p726-733).

The duration of compression is also vital. Short, intermittent loading improves the proliferation of cells (Rubin et al., 1984, p397-402) whereas large numbers of cycles enhance synthesis of proteoglycans (Chowdhury et al., 2003, p105-111). GAG synthesis is stimulated by dynamic compression with a low force, which could be improved with cyclic compressions (Larsson et al., 1991, p388-394). The amount of ECM collected raises with increased culture duration in dynamic compression models (Mauck et al., 2000, p252–260). Also, dynamic load application when growth factors with high molecular weights are present, stimulates mechanical and chemical environment for optimizing tissue growth (Chahine et al., 2009, p968-975).

Integrin and TGFβ modulate the changes caused by compression. In the studies performed by Chowdhury et al., TGFβ had stimulatory and α5β1 integrin had modulatory effects; but, presence of a peptide inhibited cell proliferation and proteoglycan synthesis under the dynamic compression (Chowdhury et al., 2004, p873-881). Dynamic compression leads to inhibition

13

of COX-2 and iNOS expression together with nitric oxide and PGE_2 release (Chowdhury et al., 2001, p1168-1174).

To sum up, understanding all these varying conditions affecting the cell proliferation and investigation of optimal conditions is vital for creating successful tissue engineered constructs in order to repair the cartilage.

One of the greatest challenges for three-dimensional tissue engineering products is heterogeneous nutrient transport limitation. Perfusion or mechanical stimulation could be used to transport nutrients and waste products. This problem could be resolved by production of bioreactors answering the specific needs of the chondrocyte metabolism.

A bioreactor system designed by Bader et al. for perfusion of fluid through the agarose constructs in cylindrical shape achieved a very important DNA and GAG increase in the core of three-dimensional constructs (Bader et al., 2009, p417-437). Bioreactor systems could be used in the control of oxygen and carbon dioxide concentrations, pH, temperature and nutrients through diffusion, osmosis and perfusion (Chowdhury, 2011c).

All these circumstances could be carefully selected and created by a bioreactor with compressive applications in order to enhance the cell growth. In order to improve the cell viability in the core, nutrient and waste transport to the core of the construct should be ensured. Application of dynamic loading to increase transportation is a solution for this condition.

When glucose amount decreases, chondrocytes start respiring aerobically, consuming oxygen. Therefore, monitoring glucose and oxygen are significant. Fluorescence methods could be used in monitoring of the molecular transportation. Application of dynamic strain improves the transportation process and anaerobic functions whereas static strain application inhibits the transportation (Chowdhury, 2011c). Perfusion cultures have the capacity to support higher cell numbers compared to static cultures. Also, rotatory movements improve the heterogeneity (Zhou, 2008).

New scaffolds which have larger pores for easier nutrient and waste transfer, or from different materials such as fiber (Malda, 2004) could be produced in order to increase nutrient transportation. For monitoring the nutrients and wastes, one follow-up method is the use of micro dialysis (Boubriak, 2006).

Further research area in monitoring is the four dimensional computerized technology which not only monitors the transport, but also predicts the utilization of these molecules (Ellis et al., 2005).

The main disadvantage would be the fact that the results will be based on assumptions. Supplying the nutrients to the cells as a bulk is another area which could be further studied. Automated systems with sensors for detection and feedback systems for regulation (Chowdhury, 2011c) are the new developing technology.

Also, there is research going on for creating smaller bioreactors for varying pH and oxygen levels (Brune, 1998). In the same way, microscopic techniques for nutrient and oxygen transportation are under investigation. Chondrocytes require some special considerations like removal of toxins and uniform seeding of the scaffolds (Chowdhury, 2011c). Improving these requirements would create a more desirable medium for cartilage proliferation.

Increase in culture period has a very significant effect on proteoglycan synthesis. This could be greatly improved with use of better bioreactor systems. As continuation of these experiments, a rotating wall vessels cartilage bioreactor, with improved nutrient and homogenousity systems could be used to investigate the effect of agarose concentration and culture period on the constructs.

In order to test the effect of agarose concentration and culture period on mechanical properties of the cell further, dynamic intermittent compression with different frequencies could be experimented to see the correlation between the stiffness and activation of certain cell metabolism pathways.

Cartilage Tissue Engineering Products in the Market

ACI is the most widely used tissue engineered product in the market. Genzyme Biosurgery, the first company introducing this technique with Carticel, is still leader of the United States market. In 2002, the sales of Carticel were $20.4 million (Husing et al., 2003). The biopsy storage up to 2 years and patients receiving their own cells are the unique selling points of Carticel whereas need for two operation sites, unavailability to osteoarthritis patients and old people are the disadvantages.

Tissue removed from non-load bearing sections are harvested for 5 weeks and implanted, followed by perichondral flap which is the classical autologous cell transplantation (Carticel, 2012). It is the most expensive product in the UK by the price £4000-5000 (NICE, 2008).

Genzyme acquired Verigen and merged the advantages of collagen membrane, matrix-induction and minimal-invasion to its technology (Husing et al., 2003).

Bio-Tissue Technologies applies arthroscopic grafts for mechanical stability by Bioseed-C. Stability, single operation, trauma and degeneration repair, short culture time of 3 weeks, three dimensional shape design for damaged area, biodegradability and flexibility are the advantages. However, long scaffold degradation time requires patient coherence (Biotissue, 2012).

TETEC targets defects such as meniscal tears and intervertebral disc lesions as well as weight-bearing joints by NOVOCART (Husing et al., 2003). Biphasic matrix allowing physiological cell distribution and short culture time are advantages whereas the product not being compatible with degenerative conditions, the treatment being dependent on the healthy inner cartilage structures and maximum 14cm^3 defect size are the disadvantages (Novocart, 2011).

TiGenix owns the first European Union approved product Chondrocelect which uses adult stem cells. Using biological collagen membrane is an advantage. This procedure is only available for femoral chondyle in adults (Husing et al., 2003; Tigenix, 2012). Tigenix acquired Orthomimetics with its resorbable Chondromimetics product aiming small defects.

Co.don, by chondrosphere treatment, aims the spherical development of chondrocytes producing extracellular matrix beneficial for 3D structure formation (Co.don, 2012).

Ormed has a unique selling point of providing training and follow up products for their porcine derived collagen covered transplants (Husing et al., 2003).

CellGenix provides CartiGro autologous cell transplantation with collagen membrane as well (Stuart, 2009).

CellCoTec, with cell replacement technology INSTRUCT, provides cartilage lesion repair in a single procedure with reduced rehabilitation. Faster hyaline formation and effective results were observed compared to ACI (CellCoTec, 2006).

Arthro Kinetics provides a cartilage regeneration system, CaReS for large defects by embedding collagen type-1 matrix in chondrocytes (Arthro Kinetics, 2012). This improves nourishment, cell viability, adherence and decreased surrounding tissue damage making surgery easier. Small defect size, healthy ligaments and meniscus, young age, healthy surrounding cartilage are the requirements and this product could not be used with osteoarthritis (Arthro Kinetics, 2012).

Other companies like RTI biologics provide fresh allograft storage and ProChon Biotech, by fibroblast growth factor, expands cartilage cells scattered in a 3D matrix in the autologous cartilage regeneration system called BioCart (Stuart, 2009).

Smith and Nephew created the Durolane hyaluronic acid gel injection which offers a short, drug and pain free osteoarthritis treatment with restoring viscoelastic and lubricating knee properties. Safety, single injection together with restoring joint function, treating osteoarthritis are advantages whereas animal source, needing repetition in time, not being permanent are disadvantages for consumers (Smith and Nephew, 2012).

Hyalograft C, a combined Advanced Therapy Medicinal Product, is widely preferred in Europe. 3D cell arrangement and HYAFF based scaffold improving adhesion are the advantages. It is only used in full-thickness defects caused by trauma or osteochondritis dissecans (Tognana, 2007; Anika Therapeutics, 2012).

Osiris Therapeutics aims production of the transplantation products from the mesenchymal stem cells which has a high infant regeneration rate (Osiris Therapeutics, 2012). Other products in sector are BST-CarGel which solidifies after mixing with blood and injection and Cartilix; both improve adherence by chitosan ingredient (Stuart, 2009).

Mechanisms Underlying Cartilage Tissue Engineering

Articular cartilage stands for repetitive, cyclic, static compressive forces especially in the lower limbs; therefore, the organization is important. Going deep in the articular cartilage, chondrocyte amount decreases whereas metabolic activity increases (Schulz and Bader, 2007).

In cell source selection, the age and deformation are important since the old and deformed chondrocytes have a decreased response to biological or physical stimuli and cytokines. Therefore, chondrocytes from non-weight bearing areas of the body are preferred as cell sources. Due to limited chondrocyte amount in body, stem cells are also under interest (Kim and Han, 2000; Saltzman et al., 2004).

Bone marrow stromal cells can expand in monolayer cultures without differentiating which means very small numbers can yield sufficient chondrocytes for repairing larger defected areas and when optimum environmental conditions are provided, could differentiate to provide chondrocytes (Pittenger et al., 1999).

Implantation of matrix is also important for stimulating growth, adhesion (Captan et al., 1997). Scaffolds are used for maintaining the phenotype and proliferation of the differentiated chondrocytes without losing function (Ting et al., 1998; Kim and Han, 2000). Synthetic, biological or polymer scaffolds (Ochi et al., 2001, p172-179) could improve the stability of the product making it feasible for cell attachment in implantation.

TGFβ1 and FGF-2 growth factors enhance proliferation and re-differentiation capability in a three dimensional environment (Blitterswijk et al., 2005). The scaffolds need to be biodegradable, non-toxic and degrade as chondrogenesis takes place. Porosity is significant in providing space for growth and maintaining strength (Palsson and Bhatia, 2004).

Easily reproducible and cost effective three dimensional alginate or agarose constructs allow spherical cell phenotype formation as well as preserving the load-bearing functions and extracellular matrix synthesis but interactions within the matrix would be lost (Lee and Bader, 1995, p828-835; Chowdhury, 2011). Fibrin, alginate, agarose, chitosan and hyaluronan are the natural biomaterials for scaffolds (Chang et al., 2005).

Chondrocytes regularly experience loading therefore a gel or liquid matrix which can solidify in-vivo would assist them in bearing load and if the porosity is too high, stiffness would be affected (Kim and Han, 2000). In order to improve attachment, collagen type-2 or poly-L-lysine could be used as a cover (Grande et al., 1997). Matrix coupled autologous transplant using hydrogels with collagen type-1 or hydroxyapatite is widely used in surgery nowadays (Behrens et al., 2006, p194-202).

Mechanotransduction influences signalling pathways affecting cell proliferation and matrix synthesis by biological and mechanical stimuli. Dynamic compression enhances cell proliferation and extracellular matrix synthesis (proteoglycan synthesis).

Frequency is important for proteoglycan synthesis whereas cell proliferation takes place independent of frequency (Lee and Bader, 1997, p181-188; Chowdhury, 2011). Dynamic compression increases proliferation of superficial chondrocytes and proteoglycan synthesis of deep chondrocytes (Lee et al., 1998, p726-733; Chowdhury, 2011). Increasing numbers of loading cycles has a positive effect on proteoglycan synthesis but cell proliferation increases by intermittent short durations of loading (Chowdhury et al., 2003, p105-111).

TGF-β presence in dynamic compression improves both cell proliferation and synthesis of proteoglycans. Peptides, as $\alpha5\beta1$ integrin competitive ligands, block the response to loading so peptides prevent cell proliferation and proteoglycan synthesis in compression (Chowdhury et al., 2004; Chowdhury, 2011). IL-1β presence enhances the release of nitric oxide which inhibits the anabolic pathways and dynamic compression application could reverse the catabolic pathways (Chowdhury et al., 2001).

Oxygen concentration in the cartilage decreases when going deep. Glucose concentration is very important. Oxygen becomes important where glucose is not available and oxidative respiration takes place; in other conditions, high oxygen concentrations could damage cells (Heywood, 2006).

Extracellular matrix and ionic water content of the chondrocytes are considered to make up a biphasic system (Mow and Wang, 1999). Negatively charged proteoglycans bind to positive ions in water and total negative charge causes the inflow of water until an equilibrium is reached where the pressure of swelling and the matrix stress caused by compressive forces are equal (Cohen et al., 1998; Schulz and Bader, 2007). Extreme hydrodynamic processes can damage the chondrocytes.

Bioreactors are important for monitoring oxygen, acidity, nutrient, carbon dioxide and temperature levels in the construct together with achieving even mixing. Diffusion, osmosis and perfusion could constitute the flow of medium in bioreactors (Chowdhury, 2011; McMahon, 2010).

Product Developing Technologies

Bioreactors could be used for creating and monitoring the optimum environment required for chondrocyte proliferation, delivering nutrients and removing wastes evenly including the core. This is important for maintaining cell viability (Heywood, 2005). Good manufacturing process requirements must be met in bioreactor production (Portner, 2005).

Static cell cultures are cheap, easily disposable fixed mechanisms but parameters could not be controlled and nutrient diffusion to core is low. In the mixed flask, mechanical unidirectional mixing is present for uniform cell distribution which is good for short term use. Scaffolds could be cultured in rotating vessels (Kim and Han, 2000).

Slow turning lateral vessel with membrane oxygenator in core targets tissue explants whereas high aspect ratio vessel with a flat oxygenator aims cell anchoring (Chowdhury, 2011). Free fall principle allows low shear stress and high mass transport making this bioreactor favourable for long term use (Portner et al., 2005). In hollow-fibre reactor, technomouse and miniPerm membranes assist nutrient and waste transportation. High surface area to volume ratio increases the density of viable cells by improving nutrient transport (Davis and Hanak, 1997; Weirchert et al., 1995; Nagel, 1994).

Dynamic strain improves nutrient transport. This could be monitored by uptake of radioisotopes and fluorescence (Chowdhury, 2011). Flexercell, applying dynamic forces, and a perfusion system would improve proliferation and decrease workload in long term. Regular medium exchange requirement which is one of the disadvantages of basic systems would not be required (McMahon, 2010).

Aastrom Biosciences Inc developed Aastrom Replicell. Stem cells from bone marrow are expanded in the device for a wide therapeutical range; however, this does not provide tissue differentiation. Millennium Biologix created ACTES bioreactor for mono and biphasic transplants by allowing cartilage tissue biopsy entrance into a disposable biopsy chamber and cultivation of cartigraft together with autologous graft, decreasing the costs (Schulz and Bader, 2007).

Business Case Development for Cartilage Tissue Engineering

In developed countries, high lifespan and increased body degeneration is present causing prevalent cartilage diseases, resulting in increased treatment costs, chronic condition management duration, decreased mobility and reduced workforce.

In the world, 15-20 million arthritis, 20 million cartilage joint defect and one million knee injury patients are treated per year. In 2011, surgical cartilage regeneration market was estimated as €25 billion (Husing et al., 2003).

Tissue engineering is the only permanent solution for cartilage repair. Other treatment methods like prostheses are temporary, painful, reduce mobility and require revision. Health systems and grant companies provide financial support for extending the use of tissue-engineered products.

A grant could be taken for development of products and research in weight-bearing joints, large defects, joints receiving repetitive movements, all age groups, decreased follow-up duration, restoring the joint function and osteoarthritis from National Institute of Health, European Union Health and Project Development Sections, International Cartilage Repair Society, Arthritis Foundation, Arthritis UK, Osteoarthritis Research Society International, many universities and private institutions.

Proving and mentioning restoration of joint function, normal mobility, smaller scar and reduced pain compared to prosthesis, using patient's own cells rather than other materials, clinical excellence of the institutions and providing cell storage options highly promote new tissue-engineered products to patients.

Creating a vision as an easy, small procedure compared to bulky, painful prosthesis operations, releasing the positive clinical trial results, sharing constructive patient comments and creating reflective advertisements would improve the acceptance and sales by creating a high technology, safe image in the minds. Patient being familiar to the procedure and being less scared is important for public acceptance of products. Patient information leaflets, GP advertisements, hospital brochures and mass media could be used to familiarise patients with products and increase acceptance within the community.

Clinical Problems Related to Cartilage

Traumatic, degenerative, iatrogenic or inflammatory conditions can cause cartilage damage. Cartilage damage is graded as softening, roughening, cracking and loss of cartilage (McDerMott, 2010).

Osteoarthritis, being the most prevalent arthritis in the United Kingdom, causes 140.000 joint replacement operations per year (Osteoarthritis, 2010). Mechanical factors such as trauma and long term joint usage, susceptibility depending on gender, obesity and heredity, together with age can cause osteoarthritis. The effects on the body are inflammation, restricted moving, muscle weakness, joint damage and bony growths (osteophytes).

Management involves exercising, weight loss, drug treatments such as non-steroidal anti-inflammatory drugs and joint replacement surgery based on the severity of the condition, however osteoarthritis is a degenerative condition and the options other than tissue engineering can only temporarily manage the condition rather than repairing the tissue (Colledge et al., 2010). Hyaluronic acid injections could restore the function and physiology of joints in osteoarthritis patients for a limited time (Smith and Nephew, 2012).

Articular cartilage of the weight bearing joints is exposed to movement and degeneration resulting in traumatic lesions and cartilage defects creating pain and mobility loss. Sudden accidents, especially blunt trauma cause 10.000

cartilage damage cases needing treatment per year in the United Kingdom (NHS Choices, 2009).

Trauma could cause partial or full thickness cartilage injuries. Full thickness cartilage defects involve chondral and subchondral layers and repair is attained by fibrocollagenous tissue filling. Partial thickness cartilage injuries are superficial defects that cannot heal impulsively (Robert, 2002) due to the absence of blood supply. Besides conventional measures, Pridie drilling, arthroplasty and micro fractures promote fibrocollagenous tissue formation but also cause increased injury vulnerability and premature osteoarthritis due to abundant collagen type-1 whereas ACT provides a solution for restoring hyaline cartilage and joint function (Buckwalter and Mankin, 1998).

Acknowledgements

I would like to express my thankfulness to a cutting edge engineering researcher, one of the pioneers in the cartilage tissue engineering field, my lecturer Tina Chowdhury for providing me this project to work on and teaching me very valuable information about cartilage tissue engineering.

I would like to thank my mother Assoc.Prof.Dr.Bahire Efe Özad, my father Ali Ozad, my brother Murat Ozad, my grandmothers Müsteyde Ozad (late), Ülvan Efe and, my grandfathers Murad Husnu Ozad (late) and Fadıl Efe, for their love, care and support not only during this project, but also throughout my whole life.

References

Amit M et al., (2000), Clonally derived human embryonic stem cell lines maintain pluripotency and proliferative potential for prolonged periods of culture, Dev Biol., 227(2), p271-278.

Anika Therapeutics, (2012), Online Resource, Last Accessed: 11 January 2012 16:00, http://www.anikatherapeutics.com/products/Orthobiologics/hyalograft.html.

Arthro Kinetics, (2012), Cares 1s, Online Resource, Last Accessed: 11 January 2011 13:23, http://www.arthro-kinetics.com/en/taxonomy/term/8.

Bader DL et al., (2009), The development of a bioreactor to perfuse radially-confined hydrogel constructs: design and characterization of mass transport properties, Biorheology, 46(5), p417-37.

Behrens P et al., (2006), Matrix-associated autologous chondrocyte transplantation/ implantation (MACT/MACI)–5-year follow-up, Knee, 13, p194–202.

Behrens PP, (2005), "Matrixgekoppelte Mikrofrakturierung" Arthroskopie 18 (3), p193–197.

Benya PD, Shaffer JD, (1982) Dedifferentiated chondrocytes reexpress the differentiated collagen phenotype when cultured in agarose gels, Cell, 30(1), p215-224.

Biotissue, (2012), Online Resource, last Accessed: 11 January 2012 14:29, http://www.biotissue.de/en-ProductsPatientsBioSeedCIntroduction.html.

Blitterswijk CV et al., (2005), Tissue Engineering, p537-539, Elsevier.

Boubriak OA et al., (2006), Monitoring of metabolite gradients in tissue-engineered constructs, *J. R. Soc. Interface* 22 October 2006 vol. 3 no. 10, p637-648.

Boyan BD, et al., (1999), Bone and cartilage tissue engineering, Clin Plast Surg., 26, p629–645.

Brittberg M et al., (1994), Treatment of deep cartilage defects in the knee with autologous chondrocyte transplantation, In: New England Journal of Medicine 331, p889-895.

Brune A, (1998), Termite guts: the world's smallest bioreactors, Elsevier.

Bücheler M, (2002), Tissue Engineering in der Hals-Nasen-Ohrenheilkunde, Kopfund Halschirurgie, In: Laryngo-Rhino-Otol 81, No. 1, p61-80.

Buckwalter JA and Mankin HJ, (1998), Articular cartilage repair and transplantation, Arthritis Rheum, 41, p1331-1342.

Buschmann MD et al., (1995), Stimulation of Aggrecan Synthesis in Cartilage Explants by Cyclic Loading Is Localized to Regions of High Interstitial Fluid Flow, Cell Sci. 108, p1497–1508.

Caplan AI et al., (1997), Principles of cartilage repair and regeneration, Clin Orthop, 342, p254-269.

Carticel Tissue Regeneration, (2009), Online Resource, Last Accessed: 09 Jan 2011 16:59, http://www.drmendbone.com/swedish.htm.

Carticel, (2012), Genzyme, Online Resource, Last Accessed: 09 January 2012 15:47, http://www.carticel.com/patients/treatment.aspx.

Carticept Medical, (2010), Online Resource, Last Accessed: 11 January 2011 13:29 http://www.carticept.com/clinical-trials.html.

Cartilage Damage, (2009), NHS Choies, Online Resource, Last Accessed: 12 January 2011 10:22, http://www.nhs.uk/conditions/cartilage-damage/Pages/Introduction.aspx.

CellCoTec, (2006), Online Resource, Last Accessed: 09 Jan 2011 17:26, http://www.cellcotec.com/technology.php?page=26.

Chahine NO et al., (2009), Effect of dynamic loading on the transport of solutes into agarose hydrogels, Biophys J., (4), p968-75.

Chang CH et al., (2005), Cartilage Tissue Engineering, Biomedical Engineering- Applications, Basis and Communications, Vol.17 No.2

Chowdhury T et al., (2001), Dynamic compression inhibits the synthesis of Nitric Oxide and PGE_2 by IL-1β-Stimulated Chondrocytes Cultured in Agarose Constructs, Biochemical and Biophysical Research Communications, 285, p1168-1174.

Chowdhury T et al., (2003), Temporal regulation of chondrocyte metabolism in agarose constructs subjected to dynamic compression, Arch Biochem Biophys, 417, p105-111.

Chowdhury T et al., (2004), Integrin-mediated mechanoconstruction processes in TGFβ-stimulated monolayer-expanded chondrocytes, BBRC, 318, p873-881.

Chowdhury T, (2011), Cartilage and Bioreactors Lectures, Tissue Engineering and Regenerative Medicine, Queen Mary University of London.

Chowdhury T et al., (2011), Biomechanical Influence of Cartilage Homeostasis in Health and Disease, Arthritis.

Chowdhury T et al., (2001), Dynamic compression inhibits the synthesis of NO and PGE_2 release by IL-1β stimulated chondrocytes cultured in agarose constructs, Biochem Biophys Res Commun 285 p1168-1174.

Chowdhury T et al., (2003), Temporal regulation of chondrocyte metabolism in agarose constructs subjected to dynamic compression, *Arch Biochem Biophys*, 417(1), p105-111.

Chowdhury T, (2011b), Tissue Engineering Practicals Handout, MAT311, 31 October 2011, School of Engineering, Queen Mary University of London.

Chowdhury T, (2011c), Cartilage and Bioreactor Lecture Notes, Tissue Engineering 3 (MAT 311), Queen Mary University of London.

Chowdhury T et al., (2008), Signal transduction pathways involving p38 MAPK, JNK, NFkB and AP-1 influences the response of chondrocytes cultured in agarose constructs to IL-1b and dynamic compression, Infamm Res 57(7), p306-13.

Co.don, (2012), Online Resource, Last Accessed: 09 Jan 2011 16:41, http://www.codon.de/.

Cohen NP et al., (1998), Composition and dynamics of articular cartilage: structure, function, and maintaining.

Colledge NR et al., (2010), Davidson's Princples and Practice of Medcine, p1083-1088, Elsevier

Das P et al., (1997), Nitric oxide and G proteins mediate the response of bovine articular chondrocytes to fluid-induced shear," Journal of Orthopaedic Research, vol. 15, no. 1, p 87–93.

Davis JM and Hanak JA, (1997), Hollow fibre cell culture, Methods Mol. Biol., Vol 75, p77-89.

Dillon GP et al., (1998), The influence of physical structure and charge on neurite extension in a 3D hydrogel scaffold, Polymers for Tissue Engineering, p375-395, VSP.

Elisseeff J and Ma PX, (2005), Scaffolding In Tissue Engineering, Boca Raton: CRC, ISBN 1-57444-521-9.

Ellis M et al., (2005), Chauduri J. and Al-Rubeai M., (2005), Bioreactors for Tissue Engineering, p1-18, Springer.

Freed LE et al., (1994), Biodegradable polymer scaffolds for tissue engineering, Biotechnology (NY), 12, p689-693.

Grande DA et al., (1997), Evaluation of matrix scaffolds for tissue engineering of articular cartilage grafts, J Biomed Mater Res, 34, p211-220.

Grodzinsky AJ et al., (2000), Cartilage tissue remodelling in response to mechanical forces. Annu Rev Biomed Eng 2, p691-713.

Guilak F et al., (2003), Functional Tissue Engineering, Springer.

Hausser H and Fussenegger M, (2007), Tissue Engineering, p237-249 Second Edition, Humana Press.

Heywood HK et al., (2004), Cellular Utilization Determines Viability and Matrix Distribution Profiles in Chondrocyte-Seeded Alginate Constructs, J Cell Physiol, Volume 10, Number 9/10, 2004.

Heywood HK et al., (2005), Nutrient utilization by bovine articular chondrocytes: a combined experimental and theoretical approach, J. Biomech. Eng, Volume 127, Issue 5, p758.

Heywood HK et al., (2006), Rate of oxygen consumption by isolated articular chondrocytes is sensitive to medium glucose concentration, Journal of Cellular Physiology, Volume 206, Issue 2, p402–410.

Histogenics, Neocart, (2012), http://www.histogenics.com/products/neocart/.

Hooke R, (1665), Micrographia, or some physiological descriptions of minute bodies made by magnifying glasses with observations and inquiries thereupon, London, England: Royal Society.

Hunziker EB, (2002), Articular cartilage repair: basic science and clinical progress, A review of the current status and prospects, Osteoarthritis Cartilage, 10, p432-463.

Husing B et al., (2003), Human Tissue Engineered Products –Today's Markets and Future Prospects, Fraunhofer Institute for Systems and Innovation Research, Karlsruhe, Germany.

Indiana Medicine, Virtual Microscopy, (2011), Online resource, Last Accessed: 15 December 2011 13:55, http://medsci.indiana.edu/a215/virtualscope/docs/chap4_1.htm.

Kim HK et al., (1991), The potential for regeneration of articular cartilage in defects created by chondral shaving and subchondral abrasion, An experimental investigation in rabbits, J Bone Joint Surg Am, 73, p1301–1315.

Kim HW and Han CD, (2000), An Overview of Cartilage Tissue Engineering, Yosei Medical Journal, Vol.41, No.6, Page 766-773.

Knight MM, (2002), Biochim Biophys Acta 1570(1), p1-8.

Kuhnel W, (2003), Color Atlas of Cytology, Histology and Microscopic Anatomy, p193, Thieme.

Kuo CK et al., (2006), Cartilage tissue engineering: it's potential and uses, Curr Opin Rheumatol., 18(1), p64-73.

Larsson T et al., (1991), Cartilage Matrix Proteins, Matrix 11, p388–394.

Lee DA, Bader DL, (1997), Compressive strains at physiological frequencies influence the metabolism of chondrocytes seeded in agarose. J Orthop Res.15 p181–8.

Lee DA and Bader DL, (1995), The development and characterization of an in vitro system to study strain induced cell deformation in isolated chondrocytes, In Vitro Cell Dev Biol Anim., 31(11), p828-35.

Lee DA et al., (1998), Dynamic mechanical compression influences nitric oxide production by articular chondrocytes seeded in agarose, J. Orth. Res.16, p726-733.

Loeb L, (1897) Uber die Entstehung von Bindegewebe, Leukocyten und roten Blutkorperchen aus Epithel und uber eine Methode, isolierte Gewebsteile zu zuchten, Stern.

Malda J et al., (2004), The effect of PEGT/PBT scaffold architecture on oxygen gradients in tissue engineered cartilaginous constructs, Biomaterials. Vol25, Issue 6, p5773-5780.

Marieb EN and Hoehn K, (2009), Human Anatomy and Physiology, p131-133, International Edition, Benjamin Cummings- Pearson.

Mauck RL et al., (2000), Functional tissue engineering of articular cartilage through dynamic loading of chondrocyte-seeded agarose gels, J. Biomech. Eng. 122, p252–260.

McDerMott I, (2010),Cartilage Damage, Sports Orthopaedics UK, Online Resource, Last Accessed: 12 January 2011 10:48, http://www.sportsortho.co.uk/article.asp?article=60.

McMahona LA et al., (2010), Chapter 4, The state-of-the-art in cartilage bioreactors.

Mow VC and Wang CC, (1999), Some bioengineering considerations for tissue engineering of articular cartilage, Clin Orthop., 367, p204–223.

Murrell GA et al., (1995), Biochem. Biophys. Res. Commun. 206, p15–21.

Nagel A, (1994), Human cancer and primary cell culture in the new hybrid bioreactor system technomouse, Animal cell technology: products of today, prospects for tomorrow, p296-298, Oxford.

Nature Biotechnology (2000) 18, IT56 - IT58 doi:10.1038/80103.

Nice, (2008), The use of autologous chondrocyte implantation for the treatment of cartilage defects in knee joints.

Novocart, (2011), Aesculap Orthopaedics, BRAUN.

Ochi M et al., (2001), Current concepts in tissue engineering technique for repair of cartilage Defect, Artif Organs 25, p172–179.

Osiris Therapeutics, (2012), Online Resource, Last Accessed: 09 Jan 2011 16:35, http://www.osiris.com/tech.php.

Osteoarthritis, (2010), NHS Choices, Online Resource, Last Accessed: 11 January 2012 11:50, http://www.nhs.uk/conditions/osteoarthritis/Pages/Introduction.aspx.

Palsson BO And Bhatia SN, (2004), Tissue Engineering, p244-267, Pearson.

Parkkinen JJ et al., (1992), Local stimulation of proteoglycan synthesis in articular cartilage explants by dynamic compression in vitro, *J Orthop Res*, 10(5), p610-620.

Pittenger MF et al., (1999), Multilineage potential of adult human mesenchymal stem cells, Science, 284, p143-147.

Portner R et al., (2005), Bioreactor design for tissue engineering, Journal of Bioscience and Engineering, Vol.100 No.3, p235-242.

Robert A et al., (2002), Chondral injuries, Curr Opin Rheumatol, 14, p134-141.

Rous P and Jones FS, (1916), A method for obtaining suspensions of living cells from the fixed tissues, and for the planting out of individual cells, J Exp Med., 23, p549-555.

Rubin CT, Lanyon LE, (1984), J. Bone Joint Surg. Am. 66 (1984) p397–402.

Saltzman WM et al., (2004), Tissue Engineering, p435-441, Oxford.

Saw KY et al., (2011), Articular cartilage regeneration with autologous peripheral blood progenitor cells and hyaluronic Acid after arthroscopic subchondral drilling: a report of 5 cases with histology, Arthroscopy 27 (4), p493–506.

Schleiden MJ, (1838), Beiträge zur phytogenesis, Müller-s Arch Anat Physiol Wissenschaftliche, p136-178.

Schwann T, (1839), Mikroskopische Untersuchungen über die Übereinstimmung in der Struktur und dem Wachsthum der Thiere und Pflanzen. Harri, Germany: Verslag der Sander-schen Buchhandlung.

Smith and Nephew, (2012), Online Resource, Last Accessed: 11 January 2011 13:25, http://global.smith-nephew.com/us/product23822.htm, http://www.durolane.com/index/156/About-Durolane.html.

Steadman JR et al., (1997), Long-term results of full-thickness articular cartilage defects of the knee treated with debridement and microfracture, Read at the Linvatec Sports Medicine Conference, Vail, Colorado.

Stoltz JF, (2000), Mechanobiology: Cartilage and Chondrocyte, Biomedical and Health Research, IOS Press.

Stuart M, (2009), Cartilage repair, What's the right combination, Vol14 No.8 Windhover Information Inc.

TiGenix, (2012), Online Resource, Last Accessed: 09 Jan 2011 16:39, http://www.tigenix.com/en/index.php?id=236.

Ting V et al., (1998), In vitro prefabrication of human cartilage shapes using fibrin glue and human chondrocytes, Ann Plast Surg, 40, p413-421.

Tognana E et al., (2007), Cells Tissues Organs, Hyalograft C: hyaluronan-based scaffolds in tissue-engineered cartilage, 186(2), p97-103.

Tortora GJ and Derrickson B, (2006), Principles of Anatomy and Physiology, p129-130, 11th Edition, Wiley.

Weirchert H et al., (1995), Cultivation of animal cells in a new modular minifermenter, Animal cell technology: developments towards the 21st century, p907-913, Kluwer Academic Publishers.

Wheeless CR, (2011), Wheeless' Textbook of Orthopaedics, Online Resource, Last Accessed: 14 December 2011 15:34, http://www.wheelessonline.com/ortho/articular_cartilage.

WHO, 2012, chronic rheumatic conditions, http://www.who.int/chp/topics/rheumatic/en/.

William CS and Melissa CS, (2010), Osteoarthritis, MedicineNet, Online Resource, Last Accessed: 11 January 2011 17:45, http://www.medicinenet.com/osteoarthritis/article.htm.

Winterswijk PJ and Nout E, (2007), Tissue Engineering and Wound Healing: An Overview: History of Tissue Engineering, Online Resource, Last

Accessed: 09 January 2012 14:30,
http://www.medscape.com/viewarticle/566133_2.

Zhou S et al., (2008), Nutrient gradients in engineered cartilage: Metabolic kinetics measurement and mass transfer modeling, Wiley Periodicals, Volume 101, Issue 2, p408–421.

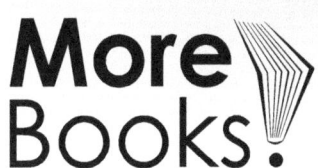
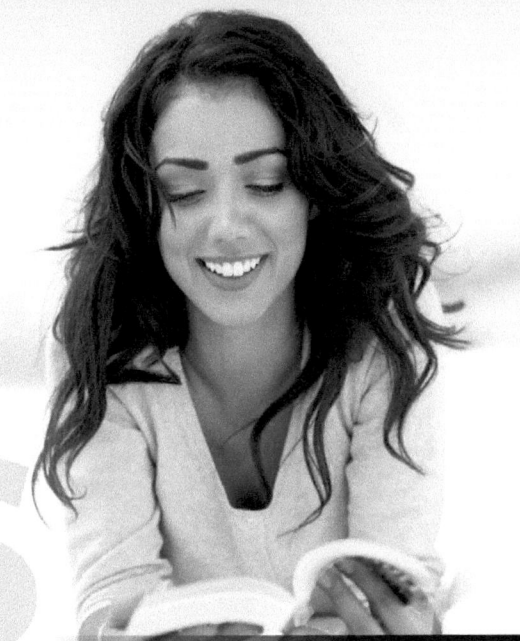
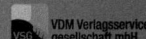

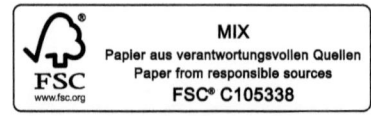
Printed by Books on Demand GmbH, Norderstedt / Germany